Heart Matters

Survive, thrive and learn from your heart surgery

Paul Arinaga

For Veronica, who stood by me through the hardest days, with love.

For the surgical team and all the nurses and doctors of Unit E437 of UZ Leuven, for the doctor's at Clinique St. Michel who diagnosed my heart condition, and, most of all, for Dr. Françoise Lambert, who discovered the anomaly in my heart and had the good sense to insist that I get it checked immediately, with an enormous feeling of gratitude.

Contents

Introduction

This book started out as a memoir purely for myself and, to a lesser extent, for my immediate family and a few friends. I simply wanted to record my experience of having a heart operation and the insights I had gained from it. I started writing the book during the first weeks after I got home from the hospital.

In the course of writing the book, however, I realized that it might actually be useful for more people. I realized, in particular, that – as was my case – before getting their operation many people probably wonder what it's like. They want to know not only what will happen in a clinical sense, but also how they will feel when put in certain situations. They don't only want to know the "facts"; they also want to understand their "feelings".

For me, this book clearly achieves its initial objective. I've recorded my experience and can now share it with family and friends. I hope that it also achieves its second objective of comforting people who are about to undergo heart surgery (or any major surgery, for that matter).

However, if I've done my job well – and you the reader are open to it – then this book also has the potential to achieve a third objective: to give you some new insights on life.

During the Middle Ages, alchemists tried to transform base metals into gold. As far as we know, they never succeeded. However, I believe that we each have the opportunity to bring to our life a kind of "spiritual alchemy". We can take the "negative" experience that we've been given and transform it into something "positive". Helping you discover how you might do this is my third objective.

Everyone is different, of course, so this book may affect different people in different ways. No matter who you are, however, I hope that you find something of value in these pages. Then I might feel that I not only have a "new" heart but also a "heart of gold"!

Paul Arinaga
June 6, 2014

PART I: The Operation and its Immediate Aftermath

Day of Days

My eyes open and after a few seconds I realize I'm back. Not back from the abyss, just back from a long night. A strange calm hangs over me like a light, pleasant mist. After a few more seconds I realize that I've landed in neither heaven nor hell. I am in the intensive care unit after a surgery to repair the mitral valve in my heart.

I'm still rather dazed by the anesthetic but conscious enough to realize that I am alive. I feel grateful. I'll get a second chance in life. I'll get to see my daughter, Leinani, who will be born in one month's time.

∞∞∞

Waking up after a major surgery is a strange feeling (and this was the third time for me – thirty years earlier I had two surgeries that also required general anesthesia). It is like nothing else. Perhaps the closest it comes to is waking up after a night of hard partying. Imagine you've been out drinking heavily, dancing up a storm and you finally get to bed at five o'clock in the morning. Then two hours later someone wakes you up. This is much too early!

I'm so groggy that everything feels heavy. Relaxed, but heavy. It's hard to move.

"Unlike with sleep, when you get anesthesia you have no sense of time."

Regaining consciousness after a surgery is different from waking up from sleep. You don't remember a thing. There's not even a vague whisper of remembrance. It's as if you've had a complete blackout. And you don't dream, or at least I didn't have that impression. In the case of general anesthesia, you're also not out for just a few minutes. Try 18 hours. I had gone "to sleep" around one in the afternoon on Friday and woken up on Saturday morning. But I had no idea how long I'd been out. Unlike with sleep, when you get anesthesia you have no sense of time. You could have been out for two minutes or for two days and you wouldn't know the difference.

Anesthesia

Anesthesia is commonly thought of as being "put under", it's purpose being to dull pain and – in the case of general anesthesia – make the patient unconscious. In fact, anesthesia has many purposes: sedating the patient, making the patient unconsciousness, immobilizing the patient so she doesn't move during the operation, analgesia (dulling or eliminating pain) and amnesia (ensuring that the patient doesn't remember what happened during the operation).

Before Anesthesia

Prior to the 1840s, surgeons used alcohol, opium or other botanicals to help alleviate the pain of operations, but most surgical patients remained conscious and endured excruciating pain. That's why surgery was only attempted when it was absolutely necessary to save a person's life, and operations were largely limited to amputations and the removal of external growths.

For more information on anesthesia, please see the appendix.

I'm drowsy and drift in and out of consciousness. A grey, middle-aged bespectacled male nurse is standing over me nudging me. "Wake up!" he says. This must be what it feels like to be in the army when it's time for roll call. I seem to be in a cavernous room. There's a lot of noise and commotion in the background but I can't move to see what's going on.

"Wake up!" the male nurse says again, prodding me harder.

I don't resent his admonitions because I figure there must be a good reason why he wants me to stay awake. I think it's so that my lungs and other vital organs can start waking up (literally) and functioning again more fully.

I have tons of equipment attached to me – tubes, monitoring devices, intravenous and other stuff. I'm like a Christmas tree weighed down by too many ornaments. One of the nastiest of these ornaments is a device that's down my throat. It looks like something they might have used in a medieval torture chamber, although fortunately it doesn't feel so bad. It's designed to ensure that patients breathe during and after their surgery.

Tracheal intubation

When you are anesthetized, your muscles become relaxed and you cannot breathe on your own. For this reason – and to ensure full control over your breathing during the operation – your doctor will most likely insert a flexible plastic tube through your mouth or nose into your trachea (windpipe).

The tube serves to maintain an open airway and as a conduit for administering certain drugs. It will be attached to a ventilator machine that ensures that air reaches your lungs.

"If you stay awake for 30 minutes then we'll take that thing out of your throat," says the nurse, now apparently using the carrot instead of the stick.

I'm extremely motivated to get this horrible device out of my throat. So I try to stay awake. How? By wiggling my toes and shaking my hands and arms. It looks like I'm doing a goofy hokey pokey post-operative dance.

The nurse must think I'm a weirdo. "No, not that!" he says, with slight irritation. "You have to stay awake, not move your body." He doesn't realize that wiggling is my way to try to do just that.

∞∞∞

Lying there in the semi-darkness, and drifting in and out of consciousness, I have no sense of time, but I must have finally managed to stay awake because the nurse removed the torture contraption from my throat. It was like having a mousetrap shoved down your throat. Well, the "mousetrap" is replaced by a very long tube; better but still uncomfortable.

Actually, none of this is as bad as it may sound. The truth is that I'm so groggy from the anesthesia that I feel virtually nothing. No pain. Little discomfort. Not even any strong emotions. I am almost as calm as a Zen master...although it's a drug-induced calmness.

Some more time goes by. A new nurse seems to appear like an apparition from nowhere. Perhaps I was dozing. She's a rather pleasant looking woman with dark brown hair and a fashionable asymmetrical hairstyle (one side of her head has a beautiful long lock of hair while the other side is short and punkish).

This nurse is much nicer than the "sergeant major" male nurse I had earlier. I'm somewhat surprised when she starts to wash me and completely astonished when she says that she's going to shave me and starts lathering up my face. I thought this was the hospital, I didn't realize it was the Hilton!

The nice nurse comes back and says it's my mom on the phone. She asks if I would like to talk with her. "Yes," I say, a little surprised that I'm allowed to receive calls. It's always good to talk with mom. She's now in her eighties but as she says later: "You never stop being a mom!"

In the afternoon (although it seemed like only a little while after my mother called, perhaps because I dozed off), Veronica, my fiancée, and Elena, my daughter, walk in. Now the circle is round. I know that I'm really alive.

It was hard for Veronica, who was my fiancée at the time and is now my wife. She waited for several hours in the evening on the day of my surgery to see whether my surgery would be successful (I mean, whether all would go well and I'd still be alive). I sometimes wonder if it's actually harder for the people around someone going through a difficult and potentially life-threatening situation than it is for the person himself. In my case, I was either unconscious or so engrossed in the moment that I didn't have time to think about anything else. I also felt more in control because I was the one who had to overcome this challenge. People around me, on the other hand, could only support me. They fretted and felt helpless. In the case of my mother, it was even harder as she was more than 11,000 kilometers (7,000 miles) away in Honolulu.

Veronica and Elena were only allowed to see me for about 5-10 minutes but it was nice to see them. Elena, who was 16 at the time, seemed to be ok. Children under the age of 16 are not allowed in the ICU. I think it's because seeing a loved one with all those tubes and other paraphernalia sticking out of their body can be traumatic for a child. It's probably not the nicest sight for an adult, either.

In any case, the surgery was a success. I'm still alive, and as the saying goes, the worst was behind me.

Unit E437

T hat very same Saturday afternoon, I was wheeled back (clever, I never thought about it but every patient's bed is a self-contained mobile unit) to my room in Ward E437 or "Unit E437" as they called it. The name reminds me of the Japanese army medical unit that did nasty inhuman experiments on prisoners of war and civilians during World War II.

Despite the scary name, however, I was to discover that my "home" for the next several weeks was populated by very kind and caring medical professionals.

I was fortunate to have good hospitalization insurance so I could get a private room. Good both for me and for other people given my nocturnal habits and constant coughing.

My room looked out over the grey roofs of the maze-like hospital complex and I had a front row seat for the heliport landings. Every time the helicopter came and went I realized how lucky I was not to have something so serious that it required transport by chopper.

I could see cyclists and a line of trees far in the distance. I would come to miss being outdoors.

Surprisingly for the beginning of October, the Indian summer was prolonged. Sun streamed into my room nearly every day for two weeks. This really uplifted my spirits.

Unsung Heroes and Heroines

Despite their many good sides, Belgians are not generally known for genuine warmth or openness towards strangers. My Belgian-American children sometimes lament how acquaintances studiously ignore them on the bus or how people eye them with suspicion when they make the smallest attempt to strike up a conversation.

Imagine, then, how completely and pleasantly surprised I was to feel so much warmth and compassion from nearly everyone in the hospital. They inevitably said, "take care" after every x-ray, EKG or other exam. I told friends afterwards that it was one of the few places I'd been in Belgium in over ten years where I felt bathed in warmth (even my Belgian friends rolled their eyes or guffawed when I said that). In Hawaii, where I grew up, this warmth is what we call "aloha". It's an ideal to strive for everyday. Anyway, I never expected to feel so much aloha in this enormous Belgian university hospital. Thank you.

∞∞∞

Being a nurse must be one of the toughest jobs in the world. These people work really long and hard, and they work at odd hours of the day. They're on their feet all day doing physically demanding labor and they also need a great deal of expertise (and thus undergo substantial training). I found out that on my ward most nurses worked 10 days consecutively then had four days off; then they worked five days and had two days off. Sometimes I would see someone working the 2-10 pm afternoon shift and then see that same person the next morning working the 6 am-2 pm morning shift. This is a grind.

It's a pity that we reward and value such people so little compared to others who take more than they give to society. Here's a suggestion: show respect and appreciation for the people who care for you.

∞∞∞

There was quite a cast of characters moving through the ward. In fact, I thought it would make a great TV series (move over ER!). I was fortunate to have great nurses (I think they gave me the A team). There was Jens, a young guy not much older than my college age children. He was young but seemed to be highly competent and he was small but was strong enough to move bigger people like me. Another lady, let's call her Els, was a beautiful blonde "super-mom" of 4 children, including two-year old twins, yet still working away and commuting 2-3 hours every day to get to work. Jean seemed to be with me the longest. His was the most subdued personality of all the nurses. Although he was not exuberantly friendly, he was actually quite kind. He tried to avoid my having to get an IV (intravenous) needle stuck into my wrist unnecessarily, for example. Having an IV needle stuck into your wrist is fairly painful and then you have to walk around tethered to what looks like a tall lamp stand on wheels that keeps your IV bag above your body.

The staff working on the ward was pretty international, too. There was a Polish lady, a German lady, and my favorite: Maria, a Colombian-American lady who greeted me cheerfully every day, even when she was no longer caring for me. She confessed to me that it was hard for a warm Latin person to live and work in a cold, rainy country. She came over in order to be with her Belgian husband. I was impressed that she not only worked long hours like everyone else, but had also learned to speak Dutch in a professional context. Bravo!

Tip

Show respect and appreciation for the people who care for you. It's a hard job and without them we'd all be lost.

Gear

As a climber, mountaineer and trekker I have a certain fascination for gear. So I was quite curious about all the paraphernalia stuck into or hanging from my body.

I had a bunch of EKG sensors stuck to my chest, an extremely long tube or two stuck down my throat, and an intravenous needle in my wrist. By my count afterwards, I had at least five or six separate punctures where something must have been attached. By far the creepiest, at least for a man, was a catheter contraption up my penis into my bladder (for evacuating urine). There were probably other gadgets, too, but I was a little too fuzzy to pay much attention to them.

All I can say is that it was a huge relief on Sunday, two days after the operation when they removed the tube that was down my throat, as well as the urinary catheter. Gosh...

One of the weirdest pieces of hardware was a test tube with a wire in it that was hanging from my chest on the right side. I wondered several days what purpose it served. It was the last piece of paraphernalia to come out, four days after my surgery. The ward doctor said it wouldn't hurt but might feel a little strange when he pulled it out. The reality was that it hurt when he struggled to loosen it (because my wound had already closed) and I didn't feel a thing when he pulled it out. This contraption was literally just a test tube with a long thin wire going out of it. The wire was about half a meter long (about 1½ feet) and evidently stretched all the way to my heart on the other side of my body. Apparently this simple contraption was to allow them to directly send electrical charges to my heart should there be any disturbance in my heart rhythm. Amazing! Who thinks of all these things?

Rolling, Rolling, Rolling

Being wheeled around the hospital was a little weird for me at first. As a healthy, strong and youngish man, I never thought I'd need to be wheeled around in a wheel chair. Moreover, before my surgery and a few days after it, I was fully able to walk around on my own. It seemed almost obscene or somehow wrong to have someone wheeling me around like I was some privileged one percent person or an infirm elderly man. But this was my routine for many days; I made multiple trips to get an x-ray, an EKG or a lung function test.

Did you know that wheeling patients around the hospital all day is actually a profession? These transport people inevitably were wearing sport shoes and looked pretty fit. No surprise, as one of them told me that they walk 15 kilometers (approximately nine miles) every day. It seems like a healthy job except that they get back pains from crouching down and pushing heavy beds (picture a small lady in Nikes pushing a huge, overweight man). One of them told me she doesn't do any sports when she goes home or on the weekends; she just rests!

This department is needed in any hospital, and certainly in the hospital where I stayed. Some patients were too old or infirm to walk on their own, and the hospital is so labyrinthine that they use color-coded lines to help people find their way around. Sometimes the lines look like part of a subway or metro system map. I'm sure I would have gotten lost without them.

Caté

The day I checked into the hospital everyone kept talking about a "Caté". It sounded like some kind of fancy Italian coffee dessert, but I soon figured out that it was an abbreviation for "catheterization".

They needed to check to see if my veins and arteries were sufficiently healthy and wide to enable a catheter to be run through them with a camera. This would enable the surgeon to see what he was doing without cutting open my sternum. Getting your sternum sliced open is something you want to avoid, if at all possible, because it hurts more, takes longer to heal and raises the risk of complications.

The day before the big day they wheeled me in my bed downstairs to the operating room. There I lay completely naked (unless you're a naturist, you're going to have to get used to being "exposed" while you're in the hospital). A nurse said she was going to disinfect me and that it would feel cold. She took out what looked like a giant paintbrush and started brushing me with a cold disinfecting alcohol solution. It was unpleasantly cold but pleasantly refreshing in a certain way. I should mention that I'd been shaved with an electric razor in my groin area and thighs the day before (well, at least it was cheaper than a Brazilian, ha, ha...they didn't shave my genital area, however, in case you're wondering).

∞ ∞ ∞

After administering a local anesthetic and completing some other preparations the surgeon stepped up and put the catheter into my right groin. It was not too big of a deal. It was like getting an intravenous needle stuck into your wrist.

Now things got a little surrealistic. I was fully conscious (remember: it was just a local anesthetic) so I could see what the surgeon was seeing on two big flat panel displays. I could see the inside of my body, veins, tissue and the inelegant hunk of metal attached to my spine during a previous operation.

After several minutes of looking around, the surgeon announced that he was going to inject some contrast fluid and that it would feel a little warm. Talk about strange feelings. I could feel the warmth gradually spread through my body and see the contrast fluid on the screen as it made its way in and around my heart. This was something like the warm feeling your body generates from the inside out after you've been doing an hour of yoga, except that this feels artificial. For a moment I worried that the temperature might go too high and I'd get fried from the inside out like some hapless bad guy in a James Bond movie. But I quickly shunted that thought aside and anyway, the warm feeling began to fade away almost as quickly as it had started.

We were done. The surgeon now only had to remove the catheter. I felt relieved...until he removed it. It seemed that at the very end he went too fast or something happened because suddenly pain shot into my groin area and I got a giant black and blue bruise about the size of a fist. Unfortunately, this one stayed with me throughout my recovery. Well, this was a good warm-up for the big day itself.

Anyway, evidently my veins and arteries were in good shape, despite my love for chips/crisps. They were able to put the camera through my vein during the "real" operation.

Battered, but not beaten

I don't know exactly what happened during the operation because I wasn't "there" (I was completely out before they even wheeled me into the operating room). I could only guess what it was like from seeing the result.

"Observing your body [after an operation] is like observing a landscape of carnage and destruction after a major battle."

The aftermath of an operation is a bit shocking. Observing your body is like observing a landscape of carnage and destruction after a major battle. I didn't even remember what purpose some of the holes and cuts in my body served.

Let's start below and work our way up. First, a massive bruised area on my right groin/inner thigh from when they did the catheterization (to check my veins and arteries the day before the operation). It looked like a severe case of varicose veins about the size of a fist.

A little further up, also on the right side, and not too far from my manhood I might add, was a very large scar slanting upwards. This one fortunately was sealed off with "glue" and healed very nicely, shrinking to about half its original size. It was from here that they inserted the camera up through my veins to view my heart while conducting the operation.

Minimally invasive mitral valve repair

Until recently, the traditional approach to getting to the mitral valve required that a surgeon saw open the sternum (breastbone) and spread the rib cage apart to gain direct access to the heart. Although this approach provides excellent access to the heart, it is highly invasive. The resulting wound requires several months to heal completely and an extended recovery period with substantial activity restrictions. The procedure also can be subject to serious complications including infection and even death.

A minimally invasive approach to the mitral valve is a "mini-thoracotomy". A three-inch incision is made through the right side of the chest between the ribs. The patient is then hooked up to a heart-lung bypass machine. Small tubes are placed in the main artery and vein of the right leg through a one or two-inch incision in the right groin crease. The heart-lung bypass machine is essentially a pump that does the work of the heart and lungs during an operation. The heart-lung machine receives patient's blood, removes CO_2 from it, adds oxygen to it and then pumps it back to his body.

Once the patient is put on heart-lung bypass, his heart is stopped and the left atrium is opened to expose the mitral valve. Specialized hand-held "chopstick" like instruments are inserted through this small incision by the surgeon to repair the valve. After the valve is repaired, it is tested. The heart is then closed and restarted. Finally, heart-lung bypass is discontinued and the incisions are closed.[1]

Moving further up the body, there were also assorted little punctures that crusted and closed rather quickly. My arms and wrists were also starting to get black and blue needle marks from all the blood samples drawn and the IVs.

---

[1] *Minimally-Invasive Mitral Valve Repair and Replacement,* Johns Hopkins Medicine.

These "drug addict" markings, however, soon disappeared.

The most painful and uncomfortable wound was the one on my right chest just under my nipple. This long, crescent shaped wound caused stinging pain and general discomfort. I didn't even like my shirt to touch it. It was covered up in thick, irregular scabs that looked like gnarled burnt French fries. Actually, it's amazing that they could get to my heart on the left side of my body from this relatively small incision on the right side of my body.

I also had two holes in my neck, one of them a pretty big one, and two holes under my right arm. I don't know for what all these were used. One of the holes under my arm was quite deep and took a long time to close and heal. It also made it a little uncomfortable to raise or stretch my right arm at first.

While in the hospital, I observed how the nurses cleaned and dressed my wounds using sterile gauze and disinfecting alcohol and I cleaned them myself everyday in the same way after I got out of the hospital.

In general, my wounds seemed to close and heal rapidly, although it did take several weeks.

Many of my stiches even dissolved on their own. It's amazing what medical science and the body can do. In some cases, there's not even a trace of the incisions.

One problem caused by the wounds, however, was their effect on my breathing. According to my physical therapist, the scar tissue, combined with the body's natural reaction to cringe or pull inward to protect itself, meant that my right lung was not expanding fully. So instead of breathing with two lungs I was breathing with one and three quarter lungs for the first few weeks after the operation. I had to do various exercises to get my right lung back in shape (more about this in I'll Huff and I'll Puff: Physical Therapy).

Not as bad as prison

Although it's not nearly as bad as prison, being in the hospital is probably a little like being an inmate. You follow a certain routine imposed by the "authorities" and you look forward to only a few things each day: meals, exercise and visitors. The rest of the time you're being wheeled off to appointments for x-rays or lab tests, sleeping, washing, reading, chatting with the nurses, or looking out the window wistfully.

You can't go outside or to the gym to do your sports. As in a prison, you're confined to the "prison yard" which is the corridor of your ward and perhaps some adjoining wards. So, you make the best of it and you train in your room and in the corridor of your ward. If movies I've seen in which the hero is imprisoned are to be believed, you can develop your body into quite a specimen this way.

"'Breaking out' is a fantasy that occasionally flits across your mind."

If a hospital is a little like a prison, then getting released is something you really look forward to, and "breaking out" is a fantasy that occasionally flits across your mind. In truth, except for the constant beeping from monitoring equipment, it was fairly pleasant in the hospital. I even almost started to like it there. The nurses became like family and my private room was sort of cozy and comfortable. Moreover, I was not really a "prisoner". In theory, I could have walked out at any time.

Nonetheless, after eight days I was ready to go home. The doctor had approved my release. I was fully dressed, packed and ready to go. Veronica was already in her car on the way to the hospital when suddenly my temperature spiked. I had a small infection so my "release" was cancelled. I'd have to stay another six days in the hospital and take antibiotics intravenously until the infection was under control.

People seemed to think I might take this badly, that I might freak out, but somehow I remained calm. I didn't get upset or into a funk. I did, however, remember the scene at the end of *One Flew Over the Cuckoo's Nest* when Chief Bromden lifts the hydrotherapy console off the floor and hurls the massive fixture through a grated window to escape from the asylum.

Tip

If allowed by the hospital (and assuming you are physically fit enough), venture outside the hospital for short walks in the neighborhood accompanied by a friend or family member. If you're not allowed to leave the hospital premises, then walk around inside the hospital. This will at least help you feel less like you're in "prison".

"Smashed" potatoes

People always assume that hospital food will be bad. I found the food to be pretty good. We had nearly every dish ever invented in the Belgian cuisine. Towards the end I could even guess what would be next on the menu – cod, beefsteak, etc. – because almost all other possibilities had been exhausted. Fortunately, I generally like Belgian food.

"'Smashed potatoes' every day for fourteen days!"

My only complaint was that we were served mashed potatoes – or "smashed potatoes" as Veronica calls them – every day for fourteen days! By day ten I almost felt nauseous when I saw them. I'm used to a more varied diet of pasta, pizza, couscous, rice, quinoa, Asian noodles, etc. One day, to ease my frustration, I asked Veronica to bring some Chinese takeaway. We had hot & sour soup and noodles. It was sort of a relief, but on the other hand I soon realized how healthy my low-sodium, low saturated fat hospital diet was. I bit into a shrimp chip and could taste all the horrible grease and salt and nearly feel it entering my arteries. Yuck!

I was researching a nice Mexican meal from a nearby restaurant but was released from the hospital before I could order it. Once I got home, I went on a cooking spree. I made all kinds of ethnic and western foods and loved every minute of eating them! My first meal of pasta at home was culinary heaven.

I hoped I would get back my appetite for mashed potatoes in time for Thanksgiving, two months later in November...and I did!

Tip

If allowed by your doctor and the hospital, bring some of your favorite comfort foods with you to the hospital or have food delivered from a nearby restaurant.

PART II: Before Your Operation

An Unexpected Turn of Events: How it All Started

After they found out about my surgery, many people asked me how the doctors discovered my heart problem. Moreover, even after I described my situation to them, some people seemed to confuse it with bypass surgery; they thought I'd had a heart attack.

Fortunately, the way in which my malfunctioning mitral valve was discovered was nothing so dramatic as a heart attack. I wanted to join the Belgian Alpine Club in order to take a rock climbing course, but to join I needed to have a health certificate signed by my family physician. I went to my physician, Dr. Françoise Lambert, expecting her to just sign the paper but instead she immediately started asking me questions and performing all kinds of tests. She then listened to my heart and said that she heard a heart murmur. Recognizing that it could be the sign of something more serious, Dr. Lambert insisted that I get my heart checked by a cardiologist as soon as possible. She only agreed to certify my health after I promised I would get my heart checked at the hospital right away.

What is a heart murmur?

A heart murmur is an extra or unusual sound heard during a heartbeat. Murmurs range from very faint to very loud. Sometimes they sound like a whooshing or swishing noise. Normal heartbeats make a "lub-DUPP" or "lub-DUB" sound. This is the sound of the heart valves closing as blood moves through the heart.

There are two types of heart murmurs: innocent (harmless) and abnormal. Innocent heart murmurs aren't caused by heart problems. These murmurs are common in healthy children. People who have abnormal heart murmurs may have signs or symptoms of heart problems. Most abnormal murmurs in children are caused by congenital heart defects. These defects are problems with the heart's structure that are present at birth.

In adults, abnormal heart murmurs most often are caused by acquired heart valve disease. This is heart valve disease that develops as the result of another condition. Infections, diseases, and aging can cause heart valve disease.

My next stop was to see a cardiologist, Dr. Vandergoten, at the hospital. There they listened to my heart, did an electrocardiogram (EKG) and looked at my heart using an ultrasound machine. For the EKG I had to lie on my back. They then rubbed gel on my chest and attached some suction cup-like things connected to wires that ran to the machine. Surprisingly, it took literally only a few seconds. After the EKG, they performed an ultrasound scan. I had to lie on my side facing away from the technician. She then rubbed some gel on my back (to improve the signal conductivity) and moved the reading wand around. It was quite funny at one point as she seemed to be studying the machine's reading so intently that she started to nod her head up and down to my heart beat as if she were dancing at a house party.

What Is an Electrocardiogram[2]?

An electrocardiogram, also called an EKG or ECG, is a simple, painless test that records the heart's electrical activity. The heart's electrical signals set the rhythm of the heartbeat.

An EKG shows:

---

[2] National Heart, Lung & Blood Institute, U.S. Department of Health and Human Services

- How fast your heart is beating
- Whether the rhythm of your heartbeat is steady or irregular
- The strength and timing of electrical signals as they pass through each part of your heart

---

I went back to the hospital a few weeks later for a second ultrasound on a more accurate machine and also had my lung function evaluated. The lung function test was quite unpleasant. I had to pedal on a stationary bicycle while breathing into a machine through a tube that was attached to a mouthpiece stuck in my mouth. The worst part was that they pinched my nose shut with some clips so I found breathing very uncomfortable. The test result was not positive; I had a lung function capacity of only 85% of "normal".

Dr. Vandergoten broke the news to me. I had a prolapsed mitral valve. He said I would probably need surgery because otherwise the heart muscle could be permanently damaged. He added that until I had my surgery I should not engage in any intensive cardio-vascular activity such as interval training. He even said it might be better not to cycle, as it can be hard to control the intensity of cycling (for example, when you have to climb a hill). I found all of this alarming. I worried that I might have a heart attack at any moment. It certainly forced me to slow down when climbing hills on my bike so that my heart rate wouldn't accelerate too much.

For a definitive answer about the possible need for surgery, Dr. Vandergoten sent me to another specialist. I visited Dr. Herijgers, cardiovascular surgeon at the UZ Leuven (University Hospital of Leuven). I liked his approach because he explained things very clearly, even showing me how the blood flowed back (was "regurgitated") from one chamber of my heart to the other and where the chords controlling the mitral valve were broken off and dangling loosely like ribbons flapping in the wind.

Dr. Herijgers confirmed that I would need to get the surgery and added that I shouldn't wait more than a few months to get it done.

So, that was that. I'd have to get the operation. Moreover, as our daughter Leinani was due in December and it was already July, I'd have to get the operation as soon as possible.

Tip

Get a complete physical examination every year!

Choosing the Right Doctor

C hoosing the right surgeon is obviously one of the most important decisions you'll ever make. In my case, I decided on my surgeon, Professor Herijgers, for a number of reasons. His being a top specialist in his field was clearly a key requirement but not the only one. I also ascertained that he would be the one performing my surgery, not an inexperienced resident, as can sometimes be the case with more standard procedures. Particularly in teaching hospitals, doctors with less experience may perform operations so that they can practice.

One of the things that most convinced me about Dr. Herijgers, however, was his approach. He was very factual and conservative. I'd been to another physician who told me quite bluntly that I should have my valve replaced, not repaired. This doctor claimed that it was likely that I'd have to be operated on again within just a few years, as any repair would not hold. He also told me flatly that I could never climb mountains again because the risk from bleeding was too high should I fall (If you have a valve replaced, you need to take blood thinners to ensure that the replacement valve is not damaged or hampered in its functioning. If you have an accident you can then hemorrhage).

When I called him back, Dr. Herijgers simply gave me the facts: international guidelines are to repair whenever possible rather than replace, and the risk of having to re-operate to fix or replace a repaired valve is 8% after 10 years and 20% after 25 years.[3] Only time will tell whether the alarmist doctor was right or not, but it seemed wise to err on the side of conservatism and preserving my current quality of life, rather than solving a problem that might or might not occur at some future time.

Tip

When faced with any serious medical situation: get a second (or even third) opinion. Then judge for yourself based on a rational evaluation of each doctor's approach, track record and credentials, and most importantly, based on your gut feeling.

---

[3] Statistics from Dr. Herijgers.

What to Bring to the Hospital

Hopefully, you won't be away from home for very long, but bringing the right things to the hospital is nonetheless important. It will make your stay there more comfortable.

My list would be:

- Clothes: pajamas, shirts with buttons (these are easier to put on and take off than t-shirts as you don't have to pull them over your head), street clothes so that you don't have to walk around all day wearing your pajamas or a hospital gown.
- Reading material: books, magazines, etc. (Include some "light" reading as you may be too tired at first to read anything "serious". During one of my earlier hospitalizations, a girlfriend gave me an excerpt from philosopher Friedrich Nietzsche to read!)
- Music: can't live without it!
- Food: food you like that is also good for heart patients (consult your doctor). I

supplemented the hospital food with fresh and dried fruits. I credit the dried prunes I ate with helping to re-start my digestion and bowel movements.

Some people apparently bring their computer with them and even work while in the hospital. I have mixed feelings about bringing your laptop or tablet to the hospital. I certainly wouldn't recommend working while you're there. Nor would I recommend compulsively checking your email every 20 minutes. On the other hand, it could be nice to be able to email friends or chat with them on Facebook occasionally. Just don't overdo it.

Health Matters: Taking Care of Yourself

One thing I realized from this experience is the importance of maintaining good health. Had I been a smoker, obese or suffered from diabetes, arteriosclerosis or other illnesses, the surgery would have been more complicated and my recovery would have been more difficult and prolonged. If heart matters, then health matters, too.

I went into the hospital in pretty good shape. Thanks to my regular rock climbing sessions and occasional long cycling trips, I was muscular and strong, and my cardiovascular system was working well (albeit perhaps not as well as it would have without a heart valve problem). And thanks to a reasonably healthy diet I had no major health problems and only some love handles, as far as fat goes.

I don't know specifically how my generally good physical condition contributed to my recovery, but I'm sure it did. Probably it helped for getting my lungs back in working order more quickly. I was also mobile and able to wash myself soon after the surgery.

Tip

Stay in shape. You don't have to do intensive sports (in any case, according to some studies these can even be counter-productive); walking, swimming or cycling will do fine. Find something that you like to do, and the chances are higher that you'll stick to your exercise "regimen". Even if you rarely exercise and only have a few weeks or months before your surgery, start exercising at least 3-4 times a week. Every hour you invest in exercise will pay back during your recovery.

Thinking Like a Champion

I f being in top physical condition (or as good condition as possible) before you enter the hospital is desirable, then so is thinking like a champion. Imagine an Olympic athlete who won the bronze medal but then had a serious accident and couldn't train for six months. If you think that such people never get discouraged, you're probably wrong. They probably do experience despair, anger, sadness, frustration and other difficult emotions. They're human beings, too, after all.

Champions, however, never give up. They may be down, but they're never out. When they encounter obstacles, they train harder or smarter or both. You may not be an Olympic athlete, but you can think like one. Your mental state during and after the operation is a key factor for getting through the operation and recovering smoothly. It is also one of the few things that you yourself can control.

I'm not just talking about maintaining a "positive attitude", however, whatever that may be. Behaving like a champion means tapping into your inner strength. It means not feeling sorry for yourself and not complaining (note: there's a difference between complaining and giving useful information to caregivers such as "the pain is a 7 out of 10"). Instead, why not focus on recovering and taking practical steps to aid your recovery?

∞∞∞

In my case, my desire to bounce back quickly (particularly as we had a baby on the way) translated into practical actions. Even during my hospital stay, I made it a point to do exercises – some from the physical therapist and some of my own invention (make sure you check them with your physical therapist) – to improve my mobility and strength. These exercises were not particularly strenuous. They consisted of raising my arms in front of me or sideways, swinging and kicking up my legs or doing deep knee bends.

My typical morning routine was to have breakfast at 8:00, then wash myself, and then do my exercises. It helped to follow a schedule.

I also made it a point on most days to dress myself in street clothes rather than walk around in my pajamas. And I rarely got back into my bed during the day unless I was feeling tired or unwell.

The following are my tips for bouncing back quickly:

- **Follow a routine**: get up at a specific time, follow scheduled activities.
- **Act healthy**: act like you're *not* a patient (wear street clothes and don't loll around in your bed all day).
- **Regain your independence**: do as much as you can yourself (such as washing yourself, making your bed, etc.) – without overdoing it – as soon as you can. Your nurses will appreciate this, too, as the more you do yourself the lighter their load.
- **Exercise**: do calisthenics, stretching, yoga, whatever helps you to recover as long as it doesn't aggravate your wounds or condition (check with your doctor or physical therapist, if in doubt).
- **Walk**: get off your butt and get out of your room. Even if you can't leave the confines or your ward, walk up and down the corridor. See if you can

gradually increase the number of "rounds" that you do.

Even if you weren't a "champion" before your operation, you can still think like one now. The more you think like a champion, the more you will become one.

Tip

Try to replace negative or defeatist thoughts and feelings with positive ones. Before, during and after your operation ask yourself: what would a champion do? How would a champion feel about this? Don't be discouraged if you occasionally slip back into negative thinking. Everyone has bad days. Be single-minded in thinking like a champion *most of the time* and eventually you will become the champion of your own life.

You as champion

Believe it or not, there is almost certainly at least one thing that you already have in common with a champion: you've probably reached a specific level in some physical endeavor. It could be a sport that you play or just a general level of physical fitness. Whatever level you had before your surgery can be the goal for your recovery. Your mind will probably accept this goal as feasible because once you've achieved something or been someone, barring extreme circumstances, you know that you can do it again or be that person again. This gives you the self-confidence you need to actually get back to where you were.

In my case, a very specific and measureable goal was to get back to my former rock climbing level and to move beyond it. The pure joy of a physical pursuit also was a motivator. I couldn't wait to get back on the rocks and climbing walls. I was "banned" for six weeks from lifting anything heavy, however, so I had to bide my time. Even when I was allowed to start climbing again, my doctor said "it would be better" for my wounds if I didn't fall. That unnerved me slightly. It also no doubt hampered my climbing abilities; one needs to move with confidence and commit to a move when climbing.

I could easily gauge the speed of my recovery because climbing has a very precise system that helps you track your progress. After taking courses and training over several years, the top level I had achieved was climbing a 6A+ indoors (a 5.10C in the Yosemite Decimal System, advanced level) and lead climbing (being the one to clip in quick draws to protect a route) a 5B outdoors. The difference between my former physique and my post-operative physique was a source of frustration and dismay, however. The first few times I went climbing after the surgery I was disappointed to discover that my level had dropped several notches.

Coming home from one such climbing session, I found myself a little angry and frustrated, and the thought of quitting climbing – something that I love doing – even crossed my mind. What helped me to continue was the knowledge that with regular training I could make a "comeback", as well as Veronica's gentle admonition to "take it easy and just enjoy it". The latter helped me put things back into perspective. After all, climbing was supposed to be fun!

∞∞∞

You will have "bad" days and experience frustration, but keep on going. Eventually, you will bounce back. Recovery from a major operation is a long process. It requires patience and perseverance. As with life in general, there are ups and downs. Try to take the downs in stride and stay focused on the end goal. If it helps, imagine yourself as a champion or some other strong character. Personally, I think of myself as if I'm a member of an elite, special forces unit. This probably sounds goofy, but it actually helps me to maintain a certain pride and standard for myself. I won't let myself slip into self-pity or passivity.

Having said all this, please remember that being proud and proactive doesn't mean being hard on yourself. Be gentle with yourself, too. After all, you've just had a major surgery!

Tip

Find people to emulate. Think of actual or imaginary people you admire for their strength of character and personal fortitude. Imagine that you are they. Do the things you imagine they would do. Respond to situations as you imagine they would respond. Use them as your "compass".

What if you have a permanently reduced physical condition?

In some cases, a patient may suffer from a reduced level of physical fitness due to complications during the surgery or some other cause. If that's the case, it simply may not be realistic to reach your former level of physical fitness. What you can still do, however, is define a level of fitness that is realistic given the new situation, and then strive to achieve it. Moreover, you don't always need to accept at face value the limits that are defined for you by doctors or others. Each time you achieve your goal, you can raise the bar still higher.

Alternatively, you may also use this experience to set a new goal in a different area of your life, whether it is your career, community, family or something else. Achievement of your goals in other areas of your life might help make up, at least partly, for the fact that you can't achieve your physical goals.

∞∞∞

Keep your cool

You may be tired of hearing about climbing, but thanks to it I was able to maintain my composure during my hospital stay. Climbing is not only a highly physical, extreme sport; it's also a mental game. It's you against yourself. When you panic, you either freeze up (I've seen this happen to someone...she had to be "rescued" from the side of a mountain even though she wasn't actually in any real danger) or you do something stupid. Panic often results in your taking a fall.

Particularly when climbing outdoors it's easy to get spooked that you're going to take a nasty fall. You may be trying to climb a difficult passage high above the last quick draw protection that you clipped in. Since there are several meters or yards of unsecured rope that means that if you fall at that point you'll take a big fall and, in the worst case, you may swing like a pendulum and crash into something. I've learned that at such moments it works well if you stay calm, breathe and use your brain. Instead of making a reckless attempt to scramble up, it's better to breathe, trust your footholds, try to maintain your balance and try to find the best next moves. This doesn't always work. Sometimes you do fall anyway. But you feel calmer and more in control.

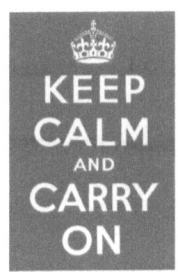

Staying cool when climbing outdoors can have life and death consequences. If you climb long enough outdoors, you will inevitably be faced with an emergency situation, hopefully one that's not too severe. Fortunately, I've faced several minor emergency situations that were severe enough for me to learn but not so severe as to be immediately life threatening. When faced with such situations you really only have three choices: 1) panic; 2) wait for someone to rescue you; 3) think of a self-rescue solution. So far, I've always opted for number three. As long as it's safe and it works, it's the best option.

What has all of this got to do with getting a heart operation? My point is that when faced with a crisis or unpleasant situation: don't panic; stay cool. Stay focused on assessing the situation, finding a solution if appropriate or simply riding out the storm. Panicking is never good; it just makes you feel worse. Staying cool not only improves your chances of making it through difficult situations, it also ensures that you feel better while doing so.

Tip

Before you get your operation, try to cultivate an attitude of calmness. You might even consider taking up climbing, meditation, surfing, archery or any other activity that focuses and relaxes the mind.

PART III: Home Again

"Now this is not the end. It is not even the beginning of the end. But it is, perhaps, the end of the beginning."

--- Winston Churchill, a speech at the Lord Mayor's Day luncheon at the Mansion House, London, 9 November 1942 (after the Allies' victory at El Alamein)

A Shadow of My Former Self

O ne thing that was shocking after my operation was how quickly the body degenerates. This is another reason for staying in good shape. Then, when you have your surgery, you will degenerate from a higher level and end up at a less low level.

During the course of the surgery and my stay in the hospital I lost five kilos (about 10 lbs.). Most of this, unfortunately, was probably muscle mass. My once muscular strong cyclist and climber legs and arms – while not necessarily toothpicks – now looked skinny. I was a spindly shadow of my former self. It's depressing how quickly the body can go downhill.

There was not even any cosmetic benefit from my weight loss since most of it was lost muscle mass rather than lost love handles.

Apart from losing muscle mass, the most shocking change in my condition was my breathing. Whereas before I could bound up stairs barely losing my breath, initially I could only trudge up one or two flights of stairs gasping for breath and worry that I would collapse at the top.

Even walking on level ground was a challenge. I resigned myself to being passed by every other person, even older people. I could only walk short distances before needing to take a break. Now I was a good match for my pregnant wife-to-be, Veronica. "Heartie" and "Preggie" could both only walk a little faster than a couple in their eighties.

Tip

Don't be disheartened by the condition of your body after your operation. Time – combined with sensible effort – heals all.

Slowing Down

Despite now being about as fast as a "grandpa" at the ripe "young" age of 50, I discovered some benefits of being forced to slow down. I didn't feel stressed to get anywhere. Most of the time I just took my time and marveled at how stressed everyone around me was. Women were the most noticeable stress bunnies because I could hear them coming rapidly up from behind as I sauntered along. "Clop, clop, clop," would go the sound of heels on cobblestones. It seemed like they were trotting along faster than a lot of horses. Men were stressed, too, but less noticeable without heels.

I wondered if I'd be able to maintain this relaxed attitude once I returned to normal life. It seemed a worthy goal.

I also slowed down in other ways. Most of the time, when I was tired I lay down on the sofa for a rest or a nap. In previous times, I might have pushed myself, perhaps supporting my extended performance with caffeine. I remember a line from the movie *Forrest Gump* when Forrest is recounting how he ran across the entire North American continent from coast to coast. Forrest, as played by Tom Hanks, says in his simplistic, homespun drawl: "when I was tired, I rested". It sounds almost biblical: "Thou shalt rest". Perhaps this is advice we all need to bear in mind. When you're tired, just rest (find a way before collapse, illness or burnout find you).

∞∞∞

Slowing down also had social benefits. One Sunday, Veronica and I went to the market and did a few things around the house, but we also ate several meals together, snuggled in bed and chatted in the morning, had an afternoon nap on the sofa in each other's arms and just sat around the dining table chatting for about an hour or two. This is something we normally never do. Even our Sundays are somehow jam-packed with activities: seeing friends, going for a long walk in the woods (which is pretty relaxing, however), preparing meals, catching up on paperwork, etc. Just hanging out talking to each other when the mood strikes you is wonderful for communication and draws you closer to your loved ones. Maybe it's good "relationship therapy", too. It certainly gives you a feeling of tranquility. You power down completely. It's what we used to do a lot when I was a kid growing up in Hawaii. We called it "talking story".

Tip

You will be slower after your operation. Rather than seeing it as an annoyance, take the opportunity to slow down and "smell the roses". Read, reflect, rest, connect with people close to you or re-connect with old friends.

Zombies

P robably the hardest part of my recovery was dealing with "zombies". It wasn't the pain or discomfort from my wounds, the nausea induced by my medications or even my temporarily reduced lung function. No, it was this feeling of utter exhaustion that – like a long shadow – was my constant companion throughout the day. Even after sleeping a good eight or nine hours I would feel tired in the morning, like I could sleep an entire additional night.

I should mention that this feeling of fatigue or even exhaustion was like nothing I'd ever experienced before. I felt like I could collapse on the spot, if I let myself, and I'd fall into a deep slumber not unlike the complete blackout I experienced when I was put under in the first place. In fact, my eyes would flutter throughout the day at times and I felt that if I let them stay closed I'd immediately fall into a deep sleep.

The only time I've had a somewhat similar feeling was when I was in the Pyrenee Mountains. Veronica and I had made an un-planned trek of 14 hours up to the Brecha de

Rolando Pass and back down after spending a miserable sleepless night in a noisy, hot and stuffy refuge. While we were walking back through Ordessa Valley in the dead of night, on the last leg of our 14-hour odyssey, I felt like I would crumple to the ground and fall fast asleep right there.

Feeling tired after even a relatively minor operation is normal. The body has received a trauma: people have been cutting you open, poking you with needles and jostling your vital organs (albeit with amazing skill).

Anesthesia is also a major cause of post-operative fatigue. In fact, a friend of mine claims that some people take an entire year to completely get over the effects of anesthesia. I don't know whether that's true, although probably it does depend on the person. In any case, my physical therapist cited a rule of thumb: one month for every hour of anesthesia. That would mean somewhere between five and six months for me. It's also consistent with what a social worker told me. She said that it would take up to six months before I felt "back to normal".

A reduced lung function also contributes to fatigue. Since the doctors cut me open on the right side of my rib cage, immediately after the operation my right lung was not expanding fully. It was a natural reaction to the pain of the incision. The body has a natural tendency to pull in or cringe in response to pain. The problem is that this reaction prevents the lungs on the right side from fully expanding. As a result you get short of breath easily and quickly fatigued in general. This situation was not helped by fluid that remained in my right chest cavity for several months after the operation. The fluid was caused by inflammation, a normal consequence of the operation. An x-ray showed that my right lung was only about two-thirds its normal size because it was compressed by the fluid in my chest cavity.

My medications also made me tired, and the ones intended to eliminate excess fluids from my body (and especially my lungs) had the side effect of causing me to have to urinate as much as three or four times a night. This interrupted sleep also no doubt contributed to my fatigue.

It doesn't seem possible to do much about fatigue. Getting off your meds as soon as possible certainly helps. I suspect that keeping to a schedule and going to bed at a reasonable hour (for example, between 10 pm and midnight) also help. Probably being very active during the day helps, too. This should include some physical activity and as much sunlight as possible. Avoiding alcohol entirely or at least drinking in moderation is also probably a good idea at this stage.

Tip

First, accept that fatigue is a natural result of your operation and a part of your healing process. Don't fight fatigue.

Follow your doctor's instructions and don't overdo it. Go at your own pace. Get others to help you with household chores and childcare. Professionally, delegate your work as much as possible. Eat a well-balanced diet. Stick to a routine, including regular exercise (but don't overdo it).

I'll Huff and I'll Puff: Physical Therapy

I'm always amazed at physical therapists. Many doctors seem to have an excellent but bookish, "hands off" theoretical knowledge of the human body whereas physical therapists seem to have a very "hands on" understanding of the human body.

My physical therapist seemed to be another one of these hands on geniuses. He did all kinds of things that I never expected: he massaged the skin around the big scar on my chest to loosen it up and make the skin suppler. He stretched my right arm in various directions to help me move and breathe better. He also encouraged me to consciously breathe more with my right side than my left side (to get my right lung to expand normally again). He taught me to do this by twisting my body in such a way that my left lung would be slightly compressed. Then it was easier to focus on expanding my right lung when I breathed.

Exaggerating in this way, helped me to get my right lung expanding fully again.

Did your parents ever tell you to stop blowing bubbles through your straw when you were drinking a soft drink? Well, one of my favorite exercises was having to blow bubbles through a straw into a plastic bottle. The idea was to make bubbles in the water. I felt half like a little kid again. I also felt like one of the astronauts in *The Right Stuff* as I tried to blow smoothly and steadily to make my breath last as long as possible (my record, before stopping this exercise, was 45 seconds). Eventually I got a contraption with three tubes and balls in each tube but by then I didn't need it as much. Blowing bubbles in water worked pretty well for me.

I "graduated" from my individual sessions with my physical therapist and got into a physical therapy program with a group. As usual I was the youngest patient. Everyone else seemed to be in his or her sixties or seventies. All we did were cardio-vascular exercises like cycling, rowing, fast walking and the step machine, and later some weight training. I suppose I could have "re-conditioned" my heart on my own but it would have taken a great deal of self-discipline. Moreover, I felt safer exercising under the supervision of a physical therapist. He regularly took my vital signs and knew how to pace my training so I wouldn't overdo it. This program lasted six weeks.

Tip

If you have the chance to follow a group physical therapy program designed to "re-condition" your heart, I highly recommend doing so. You'll feel safer and bounce back faster.

It was great to have physical therapy. With my two previous operations, I was prescribed no physical therapy whatsoever, even though both operations required general anesthesia and involved lengthy recovery periods. I think that back in those days once you were discharged from the hospital you were on your own. Perhaps I was able to recover well on my own at the time because I was 30 years younger. No matter what your age, however, I recommend getting physical therapy. It really helps to speed your recovery. Moreover, emotionally, you feel like someone is closely following you as you recover; you feel less alone.

Meds and Man Boobs

Any modern medical experience inevitably entails using some drugs. I have a love-hate relationship with medications. On the one hand, I appreciate their utility. On the other hand, they seem to usually have onerous side effects. My philosophy is: use them in moderation when absolutely necessary, but get off your meds as soon as possible!

In my case, I was taking a plethora of different medications in the hospital, and to my dismay I had to continue taking them once I got home. The only medication I could drop once I got home was the potassium supplement, an orange, syrupy liquid that tasted terrible unless mixed with fruit juice (then it looked like a Campari Orange and almost tasted like one...not too bad).

My other medications were:

- **Asaflow**: this little pill was a kind of aspirin. Its purpose was to keep the blood thin and prevent blood clots.
- **Emconcor**: a pill to help regulate the heart rhythm.

- **Aldactone**: a diuretic to help drain the fluids that had accumulated as a result of inflammation caused by the surgery.
- **Lasix**: a diuretic.
- **Avelox**: an anti-biotic to treat the infection in my upper respiratory tract.
- **Dafalgan**: a paracetamol-based pain-killer.

I became worried that I was getting "addicted" to Dafalgan so I gradually reduced my dosage and then simply stopped cold turkey one day when I got fed up with abusing my liver and kidneys with all these meds.

Generally, I believe in the natural way. I rarely take aspirin or painkillers, preferring to tough it out. Pain is a signal. It tells you when some part or system of your body is unwell. This is useful information.

On the other hand, fighting pain uses a lot of energy, so it's a good idea to diminish the pain you feel, especially in the initial stages of your recovery.

Pain can also have other pernicious effects. As already mentioned, the pain from the wounds on my chest, for example, caused me to cringe slightly, thereby compressing my right lung and reducing my lung function. So in that case it was better to take some painkillers to reduce or eliminate the pain and discomfort.

Despite their obvious efficacy in reducing pain, eliminating excess fluid, fighting infection, keeping the blood thin or ensuring a stable heart rhythm, there were two things that disturbed me out about my meds: 1) their side effects (especially their potentially detrimental effects on my liver and kidneys); and 2) the simple fact that I took them for so long (up to four months for some of them, not just a few days or weeks).

None of the side effects was pleasant, but one of the main potential side effects of Aldactone was downright creepy. The information sheet included in the box with the medication listed this as the first potential side effect:

> *"An unusual swelling of the breasts among men (gynecomastia) can appear, and depends on the dosage and the duration of the treatment. The side effect normally disappears upon termination of treatment. In rare cases, gynecomastia can become permanent."*

"Great," I thought, "now in addition to being disfigured by scars I risk growing man boobs."

Believe me, this provided a major incentive for getting off these meds as soon as possible!

Another issue I encountered was nausea. I started to have these attacks during which I suddenly felt like throwing up. It was similar to the "dry heaves" as we used to call them in college. The dry heaves are when you feel like throwing up but are not able to get anything out because you're too dehydrated. Throwing up is unpleasant, but normally once you've thrown up you start to feel a little better. This was different. This was just a persistent case of the dry heaves that could strike at any moment without warning.

I found out later that when they discharged me from the hospital they probably should have prescribed a medication to protect my stomach.

Tip

Take your medications for as long as you need to (follow your doctor's advice), but get off them as soon as possible. Don't subject yourself to unnecessarily high levels of pain or discomfort, but do try to reduce your dependence on painkillers over time. You can gradually reduce the dosage and frequency.

Sex?

In the previous chapter we talked about "boobs" so I guess now we can talk about sex.

Unless you were a porn star or *kamasutra* expert before your operation, don't expect a stellar sex life immediately after it. You probably will have a reduced sex drive, some meds might even reduce your sexual function (only temporarily...don't worry!) and your wounds might still hurt a little for some weeks after your operation. Even if your wounds don't hurt or provide any discomfort, you might be afraid to make love out of a fear that your wounds could be damaged. As far as I know, this is not a real concern (unless your partner is a sumo wrestler who likes to be on top). Nonetheless, it's probably best to wait until your wounds are closed and to be careful not to rub too vigorously against them or put too much pressure on them immediately after your surgery.

The long and short of it is that you'll probably feel too tired to be very horny. And anyway, it's not bad to conserve your energy. Your body may need it for healing. On the other hand, the intimacy of making love may be particularly pleasant after an operation. It can be nice to have someone gently stroke your body after it has received a major trauma. It's always nice, but it's extra nice after an operation.

Tip

Don't worry if you don't feel very "sexy" or have little sex drive after your operation. It will come back. You could instead try focusing on intimacy rather than sex for a while. Giving and receiving warmth could enhance your recovery and isn't intimacy the foundation of good sex anyway?

Don't let Scars Scar You

You may feel a little embarrassed or shy about showing your body after your surgery. I felt somewhat dismayed by the giant crescent-shaped scar on my right chest. Fortunately, Veronica, my fiancée at the time and now my wife, did not find it unattractive. You should also remember that many or all of your scars will gradually shrink, will change color and will ultimately blend in with the rest of your body. The scar in my groin area, for example, shrank to half its original size and was eventually somewhat hidden (once my pubic hair grew back).

"Some people find scars sexy." Some people also find scars sexy. At least it's a conversation piece. Sometimes I feel self-conscious about my scars but I also "wear them" as a kind of badge of honor. I feel a certain pride that I survived these surgeries so well.

In the immediate aftermath of your operation, be careful not to rub certain creams on your wounds or expose your scars to strong sun as that could lead to discoloration.

Tip

"Wear" your scars as a "badge of honor".

Just Sleep

Healing is really a lengthy process. Six weeks seems to be a milestone, at least it was for me. My cough finally went away and it seemed like I had more energy. But my full – and by full I mean that I felt completely back to normal – recovery took longer. Be realistic and give yourself several months. I found that after six weeks I started to feel "normal" again but that I was still very tired. In fact, this was the period of long sleeping sessions.

When I first got out of the hospital I somehow could only sleep seven or eight hours and while I was in the hospital I often slept even less. I also had to get up three or four times a night to urinate (caused by the diuretic medications I was taking to drain excess fluid from my body resulting from the operation). So, actually, I didn't get a lot of sleep. I thought that if I could just get a few nights of eleven or twelve hours of sleep I'd start to recover more rapidly, but this never happened.

My advice would be: go with the flow; when you're tired, get more rest. It's probably your body telling you that now it needs more rest for the next phase of your recovery.

Tip

If you feel tired, then sleep! Your body is telling you that it needs rest. You just had a major surgery. You don't need to justify taking it easy to anyone. Sleep and rest have restorative powers.

Back to work

(Work and work) Well those cars never seem to stop coming
(Work and work) Keep those waxin' machines humming
(Work and work) My fingers to the bone
(Work and work) Keep up, I can't wait till it's time to go home

--- Car Wash, by Rose Royce

My cardiologist, Dr. Vandergoten, said I could start working after about four weeks. And Dr. Herijgers, my heart surgeon, told me that some crazy [my word] people even bring their laptop computer with them to the hospital. I'm not a great believer in pushing myself that way. If you start working too soon after your surgery, it's likely that your recovery will take that much longer. It's preferable to give yourself the time to adequately recover. If you don't, you'll probably pay for it later. I realize that not everyone has the luxury of taking it easy for several weeks or months, but make sure to ask yourself whether it's pride and obstinacy that are causing you to work or true necessity.

If your job does not involve physical labor, you can start working after about four weeks (or even sooner, to a limited extent). If your job involves physical labor, you might need to wait a few months. In either case, it's important to pace yourself. Start with a few hours during the first week back on the job and gradually increase them during subsequent weeks.

I started working again about four weeks after my surgery. I also started shopping and cooking (because I enjoy it) during the first week I was home (three weeks after my surgery). Moreover, due to the nature of my work (it has spikes) and the birth of Leinani, our daughter, I didn't get a lot of sleep after the initial period at home. This was difficult. In combination with my medications, the lingering effects of the surgery and the typical seasonal stress it resulted in my being completely exhausted by the time Christmas rolled around.

If you are an entrepreneur like me, it's important to follow a routine under normal circumstances, and this becomes even more important after an operation. You need to systematically plan how you will gradually ramp up your activities and stick to your program. Avoid extremes. It's easy to fall into the trap of becoming a permanent "invalid" with no routine, on the one hand, or of jumping back in the game too quickly, on the other.

Tip

You can't always control external circumstances, but try not to overdo it! Let others take care of you during the first few weeks that you're home. When you start working again, stick to a routine and try to pace yourself.

I'll be B-A-C-K !

I'm not a big Arnold Schwarzenegger fan but one of his favorite lines became my motto: "I'll be BACK!"

You'll gradually be able to pick up activities that you did before. Be gentle with yourself. You may get tired and, especially if they are physical activities, you probably won't do them at your previous level. Give yourself time.

I started cycling again four or five weeks after my surgery. It went well although I was noticeably short of breath, especially on hills. I went swimming about the same time and that went very well. The thing I've always liked about swimming is that being in water seems to be therapeutic. I went climbing for the first time after five weeks and my top level was only 5A+ (previously, it was 6A+). At first I was pretty disappointed and even a little angry, but then I decided to just enjoy myself and accept that it would take some time to get back to my former level (which I finally did after several more months). I knew I would get back to my former level because I knew I could become a "6A+ man" again.

PART IV: Heart Matters

Life and...death?

In the weeks preceding my operation, I must admit that I started to become a bit somber. I started to wonder whether these might be my last weeks on earth. According to my cardiac surgeon, Dr. Herijgers, the chances of anything going wrong were only 1 in 1,000. Moreover, my relatively young age (50 years) and overall good health (low cholesterol, non-smoker, good weight, etc.) would work in my favor. Nonetheless, I started to wonder – and it's probably only natural to start wondering – if I was going to make it and if everything was going to be ok. Even good odds don't count for much if you have the misfortune of being the 1 in 1000th person!

This situation was not helped by all the "loose ends" that I tried to tie up before the operation: getting married, creating a will and testament, catching up on my administration, re-contacting (old) friends, etc. One thing I recommend is doing all these things during "normal" times so that you don't have to rush to do them during "emergencies". It's good to keep in touch with friends in any case, although our hectic 21st century lifestyles do not make this easy.

Tip

As far as possible, arrange your life beforehand so that you don't have to rush to arrange it when you suddenly find out that you need to get an operation. Have an up-to-date will and testament, stay on top of your administration, and keep in touch with family and friends.

Death: the end or the beginning?

Let's get to the heart of the matter, or part of it anyway: death. Death is something that nearly all people fear. It's normal and natural to have a survival instinct but perhaps we dwell upon death too much. When I say "dwell upon" I mean more that it is omnipresent yet just below the surface. It casts a long shadow over our subconscious mind.

It's frightening to contemplate the possibility of your own death. It's also potentially disappointing. On the one hand, there were so many things that you still wanted to do. On the other hand, you may feel like: "This is it? That's the sum of my life? That's all I ever accomplished? That's what I'll be remembered for?"

Use this. Use this confrontation with your own mortality to reassess your life. Use it to see the good things that you HAVE accomplished (no matter how small) and what you still would like to do in the future. Use it to prioritize. Start by asking yourself: what's really important for the world, for my loved ones and – most of all – for me? After your operation, how will you use the remaining years of your life, this great gift that you've been given?

Whether you have ambitious plans or simply wish to enjoy the small things in life or both, it's important to make conscious choices that fulfill you and to feel grateful for the time that you have been given.

Cultures of Death

The way people look at death is very different depending upon their culture and personal beliefs. Depending upon these, death may be regarded as part of the cycle of life, as the passageway to an afterlife or the spirit world, or simply as the end. It may also be considered glorious, noble, or dreadful. People may treat it with reverence, grief, celebration or even indifference. Unlike in other cultures, in the Western world, there seems to be an aversion to talking or thinking about death. It's nearly taboo.

Obviously, no one knows what occurs after death. According to commonly held beliefs, however, there are three likely outcomes: 1) you are dead and feel nothing; you experience neither pain nor suffering; 2) you go to heaven or hell (the latter obviously might not be very pleasant, but presumably most readers would not be heading there!) or some sort of afterlife as a spirit; 3) you are reincarnated. Without wishing to sound facetious, I must pose the question: do any of these outcomes (except for going to hell) sound bad?

My own philosophy is that death is far less frightening than living a life of quiet desperation. As Henry David Thoreau said: "The mass of men, lead lives of quiet desperation. What is called resignation is confirmed desperation."

> *"The mass of men, lead lives of quiet desperation."*

Death is likely to be much less painful than a life filled with regret or despair. Rather than fearing your own death, perhaps it is better to focus on living your life – however much of it may remain – as best you can.

Why me? Heart Lessons

W hen confronted with something such as a major heart surgery, it's only natural to ask: "Why me?"

You're sailing smoothly along through life and suddenly "BAM!!!" you have to face your own mortality, the possibility – no matter how small – that you might not make it. You might not get to see loved ones anymore, do all the things you still wanted to do, visit the places you wanted to visit and so on and so forth.

Any major surgery is a daunting experience. You are put under for several hours; get your body poked, prodded and cut open; are in the hospital for several days or weeks; suffer the humiliation of strangers seeing you naked; take several weeks to recover; and take several months until you feel "normal" again.

∞∞∞

An operation of this kind does not need to be seen only as something unpleasant or threatening, however. It also represents an opportunity. It's an opportunity to reflect on one's life, to see where you've been, where you are, where you're going and – most important of all – where you want to go. It's also an opportunity to feel and express gratitude: gratitude for the people around you who love you; the people who care for you; the small things in life like good food, a sunrise or fresh air; and simply life itself. For what are *you* grateful?

Tip

Use your experience to reflect on your life and see what you really want out of it. At the same time, remember to be grateful for everything that you have now.

Life as metaphor

You can also examine your experience in several dimensions. One of these is the literal dimension: these are the facts of the situation. Another is the scientific or medical dimension: this is the explanation science provides for your condition.

There is another possible dimension, however, which most of us rarely consider. This is the symbolic dimension or "life as metaphor".

Your illness may appear one way on the surface, but on a deeper level it may be a manifestation of something going on in your life...and perhaps even of a greater Divine purpose. Life (or God) may be sending you an encoded message.

In her books, *Why People Don't Heal and How They Can*[4] and *Anatomy of the Spirit*[5], Caroline Myss explores this and other themes. While not downplaying the importance of science or modern, allopathic medicine Myss says:

> *"Symbolic power is by far the most potent level of insight available to us. Making contact with the archetypal realm allows us to see beyond the physical meaning of events and view them as Divine opportunities to evolve our consciousness."*

"Your first step is to stop taking it personally. Do not see yourself as a 'victim'."

Your first step is to stop taking it person-ally. Do not see yourself

---

[4] *Why People Don't Heal and How They Can: A Practical Program for Healing Body, Mind and Spirit*, Caroline Myss, Ph.D., © 1997, Bantam Books.

[5] *Anatomy of the Spirit: the Seven Stages of Power and Healing*, Caroline Myss, Ph.D., © 1996, Bantam Books.

as a "victim". Your illness is an opportunity to find your true strength as a human – and divine – being. When you learn to interpret the negative challenges of your life, you will realize that each one is actually a positive challenge in disguise.

Caroline Myss explains further:

"In every situation, no matter how challenging, you have the option to pursue the meaning behind the event. In some cases, this may mean simply trusting that there must ultimately be a positive reason for what has happened, and that when and if the time becomes appropriate, the meaning will be revealed. This is hardly an easy response to have during a crisis, especially during the life-and-death situation that illness can often be. But it is the response that will bring the most power and the clearest guidance."

Personally, I believe that there is often a link between the physical and the emotional or spiritual worlds. A physical ailment is thus often a manifestation of something that is out of balance in your emotional or spiritual world. To truly be healed of the physical ailment, therefore, you need to heal yourself at its source in the spiritual realm. At a minimum, you will need to learn to see the world with different eyes, to transform your consciousness. You may also need to make some concrete changes in your life.

While it is wise to develop and use your symbolic sight, remember that it is a complement or enhancement – rather than a substitute – to other ways of looking at your illness. It is still useful to examine the facts and understand the medical science behind your illness. Moreover, an evolution in your consciousness is not in and of itself a substitute for action. While the mind is a powerful thing, usually we need to manifest our thoughts in concrete action.

Energy Anatomy[6]

Cha kra[7]	Organs/ Body Parts	Mental, Emotional Issues	Physical Dysfunctions
4	• Heart and circulatory systems • Lungs • Shoulders and arms • Ribs/ breasts • Diaphragm • Thymus gland	• Love and hatred Resentment and bitterness • Grief and anger • Self-centeredness • Loneliness and commitment • Forgiveness and compassion • Hope and trust	• Congestive heart failure • Myocardial infarction (heart attack) • Mitral valve prolapse • Cardiomegaly • Asthma/ allergy • Lung cancer • Bronchial pneumonia • Upper back, shoulder • Breast cancer

According to Caroline Myss, each "chakra" or energy center of the body corresponds to certain organs or body parts. Together these are associated with specific mental or emotional issues that manifest themselves in physical dysfunctions.

---

[6] For the full table, please see *Anatomy of the Spirit* by Caroline Myss, pp. 96-101.

[7] Chakras are energy centers in the body, according to Hindu metaphysical and tantric/yogic traditions.

My heart challenge

If – like me – you believe that everything happens for a reason, then your heart operation could be regarded as a major signal of some sort. As discussed above, to me, life is metaphor. It is only up to us to find the meaning in it.

Let's look at my own case. On a purely factual level, the problem I faced was "mitral valve prolapse"; my mitral valve was not shutting properly. The valve leaflets or flaps swung open to let blood flow from the left atrium to the left ventricle and then they swung back too far because the cords that controlled them were broken. I was dismayed when Dr. Herijgers showed me a video in which my flaps were flapping wildly out of control.

The result of this was that blood flowed from the left atrium to the left ventricle as it should, but then a large quantity of that same blood flowed back to the left atrium. Over time this could have resulted in an enlarged heart and damage to my heart muscle, as it had to work extra hard to pump blood through my body.

I was unlucky to have had this condition, probably the result of a severe childhood infection. Frankly, most people would stop here. They would find someone or something to blame or they would say that in a random universe "stuff happens".

While I admit to having had moments during which I felt sorry for myself, I tried to look beyond and find meaning from this situation. In my view, blood could be a metaphor for the "life force" variously known as *chi*, *ki*, *prana* or *mana* in different cultural traditions. Actually, it is not an exaggeration to call blood (and breath/oxygen) the life force because that's quite literally what it is. Blood brings nutrients and oxygen to the cells of your body.

In my case, the life force was not flowing smoothly through my body. It was flowing backwards. It was somehow "blocked".

Could this have been a metaphor for the current state of my life? Was I somehow blocked? Was I not letting life fully flow through me?

These were some of the thoughts that passed through my mind as I pondered the reasons why I had suddenly been "afflicted" with this heart "problem".

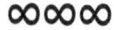

Ultimately, I concluded two things. One was that I had not been allowing myself to pursue my real dreams: to move back to Hawaii, to write many fiction and non-fiction books and to pursue a career in the field of sustainability that could contribute more to society and be more meaningful to me. For too long I had been making compromises that deadened my soul. It was like drinking a small amount of poison every day in a cocktail. The cocktail itself tasted ok. Sometimes it was bitter, sometimes it was sweet, but mostly it was just neutral. I didn't really notice the "poison" in my cocktail, however, as it gradually accumulated in my body, until it eventually reached a toxic level and had to be rejected.

I am over-dramatizing, of course. My life was not bad before my operation. In fact, it was fairly pleasant and I was blessed in many ways, and still am. While I wouldn't say that I completely loved my career as a marketing communications consultant, content strategist and copywriter, I also didn't hate it. Sometimes it was fun, and having done it for so long, I had become pretty good at it.

It was not what I really wanted, however. I didn't find creating "propaganda" to sell other peoples' products, services or ideas very fulfilling, especially when their products, services or ideas contributed very little to addressing the big and pressing challenges facing us today.

You are not alone

I suspect that many people face a similar dilemma. They are not living the life that they really want but their life is bearable or even reasonably pleasant. Not faced with a crisis, they remain "stuck" in their current situation.[8] They are comfortable. They feel pressure from their environment to conform. They need the money. There are many reasons for staying in place.

Change is not an easy thing. You are confronted with the fear of the unknown, possible criticism from those around you (perhaps even loved ones), and the possibility of losing face should you "fail".

An experience such as a heart operation is a major signal that should not be ignored, however. This does not necessarily mean that you need to upend your life, spend a year in an ashram in India or end any relationships. You

---

[8] Your "current situation" could be your career, relationships, country of residence, lifestyle or any number of things.

can also *Eat, **Stay** and Love*.[9] There is no reason per se to drastically change your life's direction. Perhaps you only need to fine-tune around the edges or to approach your current life with a different awareness. Perhaps you need to feel more gratitude for what you have. In the end, it is up to you to interpret this experience and decide what it means for you. There is no single "right" answer. However, I would like to suggest that you value your heart condition as the precious experience that it is – and not see it as just an unpleasant or painful ordeal. Matters of the heart are important, because heart matters.

---

[9] In case you haven't seen it, this is a reference to the book and movie *Eat, Pray, Love* in which the author/protagonist, Elizabeth Gilbert, radically changes her life.

Acknowledgements

I would like to express special thanks to my wife, Veronica Hertling-Arinaga, for reviewing several drafts of the book and giving useful feedback on both the book's content and its style. She's the best "reality check" I know! I would also like to thank my friends, Agnes Tarnai, Marina Kanamori and Katherine O'Loghlen, for reviewing the draft version and for politely telling me when they thought I was over-the-top and when they thought I was right on target.

Appendix: Anesthesia

What is it?

Anesthesia is commonly thought of as being "put under", it's purpose being to dull pain and – in the case of general anesthesia – make the patient unconscious. In fact, anesthesia has many purposes: sedating the patient, making the patient unconsciousness, immobilizing the patient so she doesn't move during the operation, analgesia (dulling or eliminating pain) and amnesia (ensuring that the patient doesn't remember what happened during the operation).

There are four types of anesthesia:

1. **Local anesthesia**: local anesthesia inhibits sensory perception within a specific location on the body. It's what your dentist gives you to dull the pain from a toothache.
2. **Regional anesthesia**: regional anesthesia, such as epidural anesthesia, affects a larger area of the body. It works by blocking transmission of nerve impulses

between a part of the body and the spinal cord.

3. **General anesthesia**: general anesthesia refers to the inhibition of sensory, motor and sympathetic nerve transmission at the level of the brain, resulting in unconsciousness and lack of sensation.

4. **Dissociative anesthesia**: dissociative anesthesia dulls pain and memory with minimal effect on respiratory function. It is typically used during brief, superficial operative procedures or diagnostic procedures.

What will the anesthesiologist do?

Your anesthesia is administered by an anesthesiologist or nurse anesthetist, and will unfold in four phases:

1. **Induction**: you are given medication and may start to feel its effects but haven't yet lost consciousness. The medication may be administered via your intravenous (IV) drip, gas or a combination of both. Ketamine, sedatives (such as Valium) and depressants like Sodium Pentothal may be administered, as well as a muscle relaxant to ensure deeper paralysis.

2. **Excitement**: you may twitch and your breathing and heart rate may become

irregular. At this point you will be completely unconscious. This stage is very short and progresses rapidly to stage three.

3. **Anesthesia**: during stage three, your muscles relax, breathing becomes regular and you are considered fully anesthetized.

4. **Emergence**: this is the recovery phase when you emerge from your anesthesia and slowly regain consciousness and awareness.

Once you've gone under, your anesthesiologist or nurse may put a tube into your air pipe, or trachea. You need this to breathe because your muscles become too relaxed to keep your airways open. The tube will be connected to a respirator that provides oxygen to your body.

Throughout the operation, your anesthesiologist will monitor the following vital signs to make sure that your body's vital organs are functioning properly:

- heart rate
- blood pressure
- oxygen level in the blood
- respiratory rate
- carbon dioxide exhalation levels

- temperature
- concentration of the anesthetic
- brain activity

How safe is anesthesia?

By some estimates, the death rate from general anesthesia is about 1 in 250,000 patients. Side effects have become less common and are usually not as serious as they once were.[10] There is a small risk of lung infections, strokes, heart attacks and possibly death during or after anesthesia. These risks are very small and are somewhat higher for older people and patients who have a previous history of strokes, heart attacks or other medical problems. Nausea and vomiting some-times occur after surgery, but are usually dealt with by using anti-nausea medications and not eating before the operation.

Can you wake up during the operation?

In very rare instances, patients experience what's known as "anesthesia awareness". That's when a patient regains some awareness when they should be unconscious. They may hear the doctors talking and be aware of what's going, and

---

[10] *NIH News in Health*, US National Institutes of Health, April 2011

in the worst case feel pressure or pain, yet be unable to move or speak.

Fortunately, anesthesia awareness is extremely rare. It only happens to some degree to one or two patients in every 1,000 surgeries.[11]

What is it like to go under?

Although people often compare getting general anesthesia to going to sleep, it's more like being in a reversible coma. You won't feel, sense or remember anything that happened to you while you were "out". Your time under anesthesia is a complete blank.

People experience different things right before going under. Some count down from 100 or 10, most never making it past just a few numbers before falling into their "reversible coma". Some people also report feeling a warm or cold sensation as the IV drugs take effect, but this is not long lasting. After going under, your next memory is waking up.

---

[11] *Tests and Procedures: General Anesthesia*, Mayo Clinic

What is it like to wake up?

Waking up from anesthesia is not like waking up from sleep. You will regain consciousness gradually and most likely drift in and out of normal sleep after you first wake up. In some cases, people experience vomiting, nausea, numbness or pain upon waking up. It depends upon which drugs were administered (such as anti-nausea drugs), in which dosages and when they were administered, as well as the specifics of your situation.

Here is how some patients have described waking up from anesthesia:

> *"After surgery, it feels like you have the worst hangover in history."*

> *"When you first regain consciousness, your body feels limp as a rag"*

> *"When you wake up, it's as if you fell asleep for a minute."*

> *"It's like when you are so tired you can't keep your eyes open. You know when you've sat in front of the TV at night and the shopping channel comes on and you're*

powerless to even lift the remote to change channels."

Index